OSTEOPOROSIS DIET COOKBOOK

Essential Recipes For Bone Health, Calcium-Rich Meals, And Bone-Strengthening Nutrition

DR ELIAN GRIFFIN

DISCLAIMER

The nutritional recommendations and recipes in this book are meant solely for informative reasons. They are not meant to replace the counsel, diagnosis, or care of a qualified medical expert. If you have any doubts about a medical condition or dietary requirements, you should always see your physician or another trained healthcare expert.

All reasonable efforts have been taken by the author and publisher to ensure that the information contained in this book is correct as of the date of publication. Recommendations may alter, though, as medical knowledge is always changing. When using any of the recipes or instructions found here, the user assumes all liability and assumes no risk, whether personal or otherwise. People who have certain dietary requirements or medical issues should speak with a healthcare provider for personalized guidance. The given recipes are only ideas; you may need to adjust them to suit your own nutritional needs, tastes, and tolerances.

When you use this book, you agree to release the publisher, the author, and their representatives from any liability for any claims, damages, liabilities, costs, or expenditures resulting from your use of the book.

TABLE OF CONTENTS

ABOUT THE BOOK

Osteoporosis, a disorder marked by weakening bones prone to fractures, highlights the critical role that nutrition plays in maintaining bone health. The Osteoporosis Diet Cookbook is an invaluable resource for anyone navigating the challenges of managing osteoporosis through dietary choices.

It starts by examining the basics of osteoporosis, outlining its causes, and emphasizing the significant influence diet have on bone strength. Knowing these foundations is crucial for customizing dietary habits to support bone density and general health.

The cookbook carefully describes rich sources of these nutrients and explains their roles in promoting bone density. It also discusses other essential minerals like magnesium, potassium, and phosphorus, which complement the bone-building process. The inclusion of protein is also emphasized for its role in maintaining bone structure and strength.

Key nutrients like calcium and vitamin D, which are crucial for bone maintenance, are central to the osteoporosis diet.

Expanding on these dietary discoveries, the cookbook walks readers through the process of creating meals that are specifically balanced to target bone health. It provides helpful guidance on how to balance macronutrients (carbs, proteins, and fats) to maximize the benefits of bone-nourishing foods.

It also details how to incorporate whole grains, fruits, vegetables, and healthy fats to increase intake of nutrients and strengthen bones.

In addition, the cookbook offers creative suggestions for healthy recipe substitutions so that classic favorites can be enjoyed without sacrificing goals for bone health. It also provides helpful tips for meal planning and preparation so that nutritional benefits are maximized while meal preparation is streamlined. Practical cooking techniques are also highlighted to preserve nutrient content in meals, such as minimizing salt and utilizing bone-friendly herbs and spices.

A wealth of culinary ideas geared toward supporting bone health throughout the day can be found in the cookbook's recipe section. From calcium-rich breakfast options to nutrient-dense snacks and hearty dinner recipes, each dish is created to be delicious while supporting bone strength. Special considerations are covered, such as managing osteoporosis alongside other health conditions and dietary modifications for different age groups. Useful advice for dining out and modifying recipes for dietary restrictions ensures that maintaining an osteoporosis-friendly diet remains accessible in a variety of social and medical contexts.

Apart from offering dietary recommendations, the cookbook highlights the holistic perspective on bone health, promoting consistent physical activity and lifestyle modifications that supplement dietary efforts. It also emphasizes the significance of tracking bone density and offers resources for continuous support and education, enabling people to take charge of their long-term bone health. Whether you're a newly diagnosed osteoporosis patient or looking to improve your current osteoporosis management plan, this cookbook is an all-inclusive tool for incorporating bone-nourishing habits into daily life.

CHAPTER ONE

DIET IS CRUCIAL FOR MANAGING OSTEOPOROSIS

Vitamin D helps the body absorb calcium efficiently, and calcium-rich foods like dairy products, leafy greens, and fortified foods help maintain bone mass. Protein is essential for muscle function and overall bone health. A diet rich in fruits and vegetables provides antioxidants and other nutrients that support bone health by reducing inflammation and oxidative stress. A balanced diet is crucial for managing osteoporosis because it provides essential nutrients that support bone health and reduce the risk of fractures.

Adopting a diet that emphasizes nutrient-rich foods and adequate hydration is essential for managing osteoporosis and reducing the risk of complications. Additionally, maintaining a healthy weight is crucial for individuals with osteoporosis as excess body weight can strain bones and increase the risk of fractures. #A balanced diet that includes adequate protein, healthy fats, and complex carbohydrates helps maintain a healthy weight and supports overall bone health.

To sum up, a healthy weight, the provision of vital nutrients that support bone health, and the prevention of fractures are all made possible by a well-balanced diet. Individuals can optimize their overall health and bone health by emphasizing calcium, vitamin D, protein, fruits, vegetables, and water.

AN OVERVIEW OF DIETARY IMPLICATIONS FOR OSTEOPOROSIS

Osteoporosis is a disorder that weakens bones and increases the risk of fractures. It is caused by the body losing too much bone, making too little bone, or both. Age, genetics, hormonal changes, and lifestyle choices are among the factors that can contribute to osteoporosis development. The disorder frequently worsens silently without any symptoms until a fracture happens, emphasizing the need for preventive measures, including dietary considerations.

Dietary sources of calcium-rich foods include dairy products, leafy greens (kale, spinach), and fortified foods (cereals, juices). These foods help preserve bone strength and density.

Vitamin D is also important because it facilitates the absorption of calcium from the intestines and encourages the mineralization of bone. Sunlight exposure and dietary sources like fatty fish (salmon, tuna) and fortified products contribute to vitamin D intake.

Understanding the dietary implications of osteoporosis and making educated food choices are crucial steps in managing the condition and promoting bone health. Additionally, a balanced diet for osteoporosis includes adequate protein to support muscle function and bone health, as well as fruits and vegetables rich in antioxidants and other nutrients that reduce inflammation and oxidative stress. Limiting sodium intake is also important because excessive sodium can lead to calcium loss from bones.

To summarize, osteoporosis is a disorder that causes weak bones that are more likely to break because of either insufficient bone growth or bone loss. To treat osteoporosis, diet changes that emphasize calcium, vitamin D, protein, fruits, vegetables, and low sodium intake are necessary to maintain strong bones and good health overall.

THE FUNDAMENTALS OF THE OSTEOPOROSIS DIET

The core components of the osteoporosis diet are calcium and vitamin D, which are essential for preserving bone strength and density. Dairy products like milk, yogurt, and cheese, as well as non-dairy sources like leafy greens (like broccoli, and collard greens), and fortified foods (like tofu, and cereals), are rich in calcium. Sunlight exposure and dietary sources like fatty fish (like salmon, and mackerel) and fortified products (like fortified milk, and orange juice) are good sources of vitamin D.

Lean meats, poultry, fish, beans, lentils, and nuts are good sources of protein.

Fruits and vegetables provide antioxidants, vitamins, and minerals that contribute to overall bone health by reducing inflammation and oxidative stress. Whole grains and healthy fats like avocado and olive oil also play a role in providing essential nutrients and supporting overall health. All of these foods are important components of an osteoporosis diet.

Limiting alcohol and caffeine intake is advised as excessive consumption can interfere with calcium absorption and contribute to bone loss.

By adhering to these fundamental principles of the osteoporosis diet, people can support their bone health and lower their risk of fractures associated with weakening bones. Hydration is essential for bone health as water helps transport nutrients and oxygen throughout the body, including to bones.

To sum up, to support bone health and general well-being, the osteoporosis diet places a strong emphasis on calcium, vitamin D, protein, fruits, vegetables, whole grains, healthy fats, hydration, and reduction in alcohol and caffeine use.

HOW YOU CAN BENEFIT FROM THIS COOKBOOK

This osteoporosis diet cookbook offers a range of tasty and nutrient-rich recipes that incorporate key ingredients known for their bone-strengthening properties. Each recipe is carefully crafted to provide adequate amounts of calcium, vitamin D, protein, and other essential nutrients necessary for maintaining bone density and strength. The cookbook's goal is to make meal planning and preparation easier while supporting bone health and overall well-being.

Easy-to-follow recipes for a variety of meals—breakfasts, lunches, dinners, and snacks—that suit a range of palates and dietary needs are included in the cookbook; whether you're a vegetarian, a lover of the Mediterranean, or something else entirely, some options adhere to the principles of the osteoporosis diet. Each recipe comes with detailed instructions, ingredient lists, and nutritional data to help you monitor your intake of nutrients.

Beyond just recipes, this cookbook offers helpful advice on grocery shopping, meal preparation, and storage. It also teaches readers about the significance of certain nutrients for bone health and guides how to incorporate these nutrients into daily meals. With the help of this cookbook, people with osteoporosis can eat well and take charge of their diet.

In conclusion, this cookbook on the osteoporosis diet is an invaluable tool that helps people stay strong and maintain their bone health by offering scrumptious and nutrient-dense recipes. It makes meal planning and preparation easier and makes sure that the right foods are consumed for healthy bones and overall well-being.

COMMON QUESTIONS REGARDING DIET AND OSTEOPOROSIS

To comprehend the connection between osteoporosis and diet, it is necessary to address common questions and concerns that people may have regarding the nutritional management of their condition. Common questions include those regarding particular foods that support bone health, the daily recommended intake of calcium and vitamin D, and methods for incorporating these nutrients into meals.

Many people are curious about the role that supplements, specifically calcium and vitamin D supplements, play in maintaining bone health. Although dietary sources are best, doctors may prescribe supplements to ensure adequate intake, particularly for individuals who may be at risk of deficiency. Other concerns include the effect of other dietary factors, like alcohol, caffeine, and sodium, on bone health and whether moderation is necessary.

In addition, people frequently ask for guidance on meal preparation and recipe alterations to conform to the guidelines of the osteoporosis diet.

CHAPTER TWO

KNOWING WHAT OSTEOPOROSIS IS

OVERVIEW OF OSTEOPOROSIS?

Osteoporosis, a disorder marked by weakening and increased susceptibility to fractures, is caused by a decrease in bone density and strength as a result of the breakdown of old bone. It is sometimes referred to as a "silent disease" because it can progress symptomlessly until a fracture occurs, usually in the wrist, hip, or spine. Since osteoporosis primarily affects older adults, especially women, knowledge of the condition is essential for prevention and management.

Identifying osteoporosis early can help implement strategies to strengthen bones and reduce the risk of fractures. Osteoporosis primarily affects the spine, hips, and wrists. It can cause chronic pain, reduced mobility, and a decrease in quality of life. Brittle bones can break easily, even from minor falls or, in severe cases, from simple actions like bending over or coughing.

A focus on bone health from an early age can significantly reduce the risk of developing osteoporosis later in life. Regular bone density tests can help detect osteoporosis early, allowing for timely intervention and management. Managing osteoporosis involves a combination of lifestyle changes, including diet, exercise, and occasionally medication.

REASONS AND DANGER ELEMENTS

Age is the primary risk factor for osteoporosis because bone density naturally decreases with age. Women are more likely to develop osteoporosis than men because of the rapid decrease in estrogen levels that protect bone density. Genetics also play a significant role in osteoporosis development because a family history of the condition increases the likelihood of developing it.

Other risk factors include a diet deficient in calcium and vitamin D, both of which are essential for healthy bones; inactivity, especially in the absence of weight-bearing activities; poor lifestyle choices, such as smoking and binge drinking; and exposure to certain drugs and medical conditions, such as rheumatoid arthritis, thyroid problems, and long-term corticosteroid use, which can weaken bones.

Early intervention is necessary to prevent osteoporosis. Healthy lifestyle choices, such as a balanced diet high in calcium and vitamin D, regular exercise, abstaining from smoking, and consuming moderation in alcohol, can help maintain bone health.

Proactive measures and routine medical check-ups are crucial for the early detection and management of osteoporosis in individuals with a family history of the condition or other risk factors.

DIETARY INFLUENCE ON BONE HEALTH

A balanced diet rich in nutrients that support bone strength is essential for maintaining bone density and overall skeletal health. Nutrients like calcium, vitamin D, protein, and other vitamins and minerals are essential for bone growth and repair. A diet deficient in these nutrients can weaken bones and increase the risk of osteoporosis. Dietary habits play a major role in maintaining bone health and preventing osteoporosis.

Vitamin D is necessary for calcium absorption and bone growth. Sunlight exposure, fatty fish, and fortified foods like cereals and orange juice are good sources of vitamin D. Calcium is the primary mineral found in bones and is vital for maintaining bone density. Dairy products like milk, cheese, and yogurt are excellent sources of calcium. Leafy green vegetables, nuts, and fortified foods can also contribute to calcium intake.

Limiting caffeine and sodium intake, which can leach calcium from bones, is also important. A balanced diet should include adequate protein, magnesium, phosphorus, and vitamins K and C, in addition to calcium and vitamin D.

THE VALUE OF VITAMIN D AND CALCIUM

The primary component of bone tissue, calcium provides strength and structure; adequate calcium intake helps maintain bone density and keeps the bones from becoming brittle and prone to fractures. The importance of calcium and vitamin D for bone health cannot be overstated when it comes to managing and preventing osteoporosis.

A calcium-rich diet won't be enough to maintain bone health without adequate vitamin D. Sun exposure is the main source of vitamin D, but dietary sources like fatty fish, fortified dairy products, and supplements can also help meet the required levels. Vitamin D is equally important because it helps the body absorb calcium from the diet into the bloodstream.

If you don't get enough calcium and vitamin D from your diet, you run the risk of developing osteoporosis. To prevent osteoporosis and maintain bone strength throughout your life, make sure you get enough of these nutrients through diet, supplements, and moderate sun exposure. You can effectively manage your bone health by monitoring your vitamin D levels and making necessary dietary adjustments.

HOW TO INTERPRET NUTRITION LABELS FOR HEALTHY BONES

It's important to read nutrition labels to make sure your diet promotes bone health. Aim for foods that provide a significant percentage of the daily value (%DV) for both calcium and vitamin D. The nutrition label provides information on the amount of these nutrients per serving, making it easier to meet your daily requirements.

Nutrition labels usually list the amount of calcium in milligrams (mg). Adults need varying amounts of calcium per day depending on their age and sex, but in general, adults need about 1,000 mg, and for women over 50 and men over 70, the requirement increases to 1,200 mg. Foods that contain 20% or more of the %DV in calcium are classified as high in calcium.

Understanding these labels helps you make informed choices to support your bone health effectively. Vitamin D is often listed in micrograms (mcg) or International Units (IU).

CHAPTER THREE

CRUCIAL ELEMENTS FOR HEALTHY BONES

FOODS HIGH IN CALCIUM AND THEIR ADVANTAGES

Calcium helps keep bones strong and prevents osteoporosis. Dairy products like milk, cheese, and yogurt are good sources of calcium.

If you're lactose intolerant or vegan, you can get plenty of calcium from fortified plant-based milk (like almond, soy, and oat milk), tofu, and leafy greens like bok choy, broccoli, and kale. It's important to include a range of these foods in your diet to make sure you're getting enough of this mineral.

It's easy and delicious to include foods high in calcium in your meals. For breakfast, try a smoothie made with kale, tofu, and fortified plant-based milk. For lunch, try a satisfying and nutrient-dense salad with broccoli, tofu, and tahini dressing. You can also snack on cheese or yogurt throughout the day.

Chia seeds are another great source of calcium that you can add to your oatmeal or cereal.

It is important to spread out your calcium intake throughout the day to maximize absorption. You can further enhance absorption by pairing calcium-rich foods with those high in vitamin D, which will make it easier for your body to use the calcium you consume.

SOURCES OF VITAMIN D AND ITS FUNCTION

For the body to properly absorb calcium, no matter how much is consumed, vitamin D is essential. The main source of vitamin D is sunlight; spending 10 to 30 minutes outside several times a week can help maintain adequate levels. However, during the winter months or in areas with limited sunlight, dietary sources become vital.

Included in your diet to maintain vitamin D levels, support bone health, and prevent osteoporosis, are fatty fish (salmon, mackerel, and sardines), egg yolks, and fortified foods (cereals, milk, and orange juice).

Fortified plant-based milk and supplements are good options for vegetarians and vegans to ensure adequate intake.

Increase your intake of vitamin D by having a breakfast of fortified cereal with plant-based milk or grilled salmon with steamed spinach. A variety of these foods will guarantee that you get enough vitamin D, which supports calcium absorption and bone strength. Supplements may be required for individuals who cannot meet their vitamin D needs through diet and sunlight to maintain optimal levels.

OTHER ESSENTIAL ELEMENTS INCLUDE PHOSPHATE, POTASSIUM, AND MAGNESIUM

Along with calcium and vitamin D, magnesium is necessary for bone health. It converts vitamin D into its active form, which facilitates the absorption of calcium. Nuts, seeds, whole grains, and green leafy vegetables are excellent sources of magnesium, and including them in your diet helps maintain overall bone health and lowers the risk of osteoporosis.

Rich in potassium are foods like bananas, oranges, potatoes, and spinach. Eating these foods regularly can help maintain healthy potassium levels, promoting strong bones. For instance, having a baked potato for dinner and a spinach salad for lunch can greatly increase potassium intake. Potassium neutralizes acids that remove calcium from the body, protecting bone density.

A balanced diet that includes moderate amounts of phosphorus-rich foods, paired with foods rich in calcium, supports optimal bone health. Phosphorus, which works with calcium to build strong bones and teeth, is found in high-protein foods such as meat, poultry, fish, dairy products, nuts, and seeds. Too much phosphorus can hinder calcium absorption.

PROTEIN IS ESSENTIAL FOR STRONG BONES

A diet rich in lean meats, poultry, fish, eggs, dairy products, legumes, and nuts will ensure that you get enough protein to support bone health and prevent osteoporosis.

Protein is an essential nutrient for bone health, playing a key role in bone structure and strength. It also aids in the formation of collagen, which provides a framework for bones.

A high-protein diet helps maintain muscle mass, which helps prevent falls by increasing balance. Breakfast options for maintaining bone health include eggs or a protein smoothie made with plant-based milk and nuts; lunch options include a bean salad or lean meat sandwich; dinner options include fish or tofu stir-fried.

Sufficient protein intake is particularly important for older adults because it helps preserve muscle mass and bone density. Protein works best when combined with other nutrients that support bone health, such as calcium and vitamin D.

WHEN DO SUPPLEMENTS BECOME NECESSARY?

Calcium and vitamin D supplements are commonly used to support bone health, especially in individuals who cannot meet their needs through diet alone.

It's important to consult with a healthcare provider to determine the appropriate dosage and ensure that supplements are necessary based on individual dietary intake and health conditions. Supplements may be necessary when dietary intake of essential nutrients is insufficient.

It's important to follow a healthcare provider's guidance when taking supplements to avoid excessive intake, which can lead to health issues. For example, people with certain health conditions or dietary restrictions may need supplements to meet their nutritional needs. Magnesium, potassium, and phosphorus supplements may also be recommended if dietary intake is inadequate.

For people who find it difficult to get enough protein from food alone, protein supplements like whey or plant-based protein powders can be added to meals or smoothies to increase the amount of protein consumed.

CHAPTER FOUR

DEVELOPING AN EQUITABLE DIET FOR OSTEOPOROSIS

CREATING MEALS TO PROMOTE BONE HEALTH

For those who have osteoporosis, cooking meals that promote bone health is critical. A well-planned osteoporosis diet should feature foods high in calcium and vitamin D, which are essential for preserving bone density. Dairy products, such as milk, cheese, and yogurt, are also good sources of calcium.

If you are lactose intolerant, fortified plant-based milk substitutes, like almond, soy, or oat milk, can be helpful. Fatty fish, such as salmon, mackerel, and sardines, are also good sources of calcium and vitamin D, which helps the body absorb it.

A variety of these greens can be added to salads, smoothies, or sautéed dishes to increase nutrient intake. Nuts and seeds like almonds, chia seeds, and sesame seeds also provide a good amount of calcium and magnesium, making them ideal snacking or dishtopping options. Leafy green vegetables like kale, spinach, and collard greens are also essential for bone health because they are rich in calcium, vitamin K, and magnesium, all of which are important for bone formation and maintenance.

Meal planning should also concentrate on cutting back on foods that can harm your bones. Avoid high-sodium foods as much as possible because too much salt can cause calcium to be lost through urine. Limit your intake of caffeine and alcohol as well because they can both cause problems with calcium absorption and lead to bone loss. Drink water and herbal teas instead of caffeinated beverages. If you do drink alcohol, drink it in moderation.

MAINTAINING EQUILIBRIUM MACRONUTRIENTS: GLUCOSE, PROTEINS, AND FATS

To support overall health and bone strength, a balanced diet for osteoporosis should contain the appropriate amounts of carbohydrates, proteins, and fats. Complex sources of carbohydrates, such as whole grains, fruits, and vegetables, provide essential vitamins, minerals, and fiber that are important for overall health and can help maintain a healthy weight, which reduces stress on bones.

Lean protein sources such as chicken, fish, beans, and legumes are important for bone health and repair. Eggs are another great source of high-quality protein and contain other nutrients that are beneficial for bone health.

Try to include a source of protein with every meal to support bone strength and muscle maintenance. If you follow a plant-based diet, make sure you are getting enough legumes, nuts, seeds, and soy products.

Additionally, monounsaturated fats, which are found in olive oil, avocados, and nuts, are important for overall health. Use olive oil for cooking and dressings, add avocado to salads and sandwiches, and snack on a handful of nuts to incorporate these healthy fats into your diet.

Omega-3 fatty acids, found in fatty fish, flaxseeds, and walnuts, have anti-inflammatory properties that can benefit bone health.

INCLUDING VEGETABLES AND FRUITS

A diverse range of colorful fruits and vegetables should be a part of your diet to ensure a broad spectrum of nutrients. Fruits and vegetables are important parts of a bone-healthy diet because they offer a wide array of vitamins, minerals, and antioxidants. Vitamin C, which is abundant in citrus fruits, strawberries, and bell peppers, is crucial for the formation of collagen, which is a vital component of bone tissue.

Fruits such as oranges, grapefruits, and pineapples not only provide vitamin C but also aid in the absorption of calcium and other nutrients that are vital for bone health. Vegetables such as broccoli, Brussels sprouts, and cauliflower are rich in vitamin K, which is important for bone health as it helps in the binding of calcium to the bone matrix.

Eat a variety of foods, from salads and smoothies to soups and stir-fries, to make the most of the bone-supporting nutrients found in dark, leafy greens like kale, spinach, and Swiss chard. Consistently consuming a wide variety of fruits and vegetables will help guarantee that your body gets the nutrients it needs to support and maintain strong bones.

WHOLE GRAINS: THEIR ADVANTAGES

Foods like brown rice, quinoa, oats, and whole wheat products are excellent choices. Whole grains provide magnesium and phosphorus, which are crucial for bone formation and maintenance. Whole grains retain their bran and germ, which contain valuable vitamins, minerals, and fiber. Whole grains are an important part of an osteoporosis diet.

Whole-grain bread and pasta can be used in sandwiches and main dishes, providing a nutrient-dense substitute for their refined counterparts. Regular consumption of whole grains helps to maintain a healthy weight and provides sustained energy throughout the day.

You can start your day with a bowl of oatmeal topped with fresh fruits and nuts or have a quinoa salad with vegetables and a lean protein for lunch.

Moreover, whole grains have a lower glycemic index than refined grains, which helps to maintain stable blood sugar levels. This is important because high blood sugar levels can lead to increased calcium loss through urine, which can negatively impact bone density. Whole grains also contain fiber, which is good for digestive health and aids in the absorption of nutrients essential for bone health.

THE FUNCTION OF GOOD FATS IN BONE HEALTH

Omega-3 fatty acids, which are present in fatty fish like salmon, mackerel, and sardines, are especially beneficial. These fats help reduce inflammation, which can otherwise lead to bone loss and weaken the skeletal system. Include fatty fish in your meals at least twice a week to reap these benefits. Healthy fats are essential for maintaining bone health.

This is especially true because they have anti-inflammatory qualities and aid in the absorption of fat-soluble vitamins like vitamin D.

Apart from omega-3 fatty acids, foods high in monounsaturated fats—found in avocados, nuts, and olive oil—also contribute to bone health by enhancing the absorption of calcium and overall bone mineral density. You should use olive oil as your main cooking oil and as a foundation for salad dressings; you should also add avocado slices to salads and sandwiches, and you should incorporate a variety of nuts, such as almonds, walnuts, and cashews, into your snacks and meals.

Finally, steer clear of trans fats and minimize saturated fats, as these can impair bone health by causing inflammation and hindering the absorption of vital nutrients. Instead, concentrate on obtaining healthy fats from natural sources for your diet, which will support bone health and improve overall health by lowering the risk of chronic illnesses and heart health.

CHAPTER FIVE

COOKING METHODS THAT PROMOTE BONE HEALTH

TECHNIQUES TO PRESERVE NUTRIENTS WHILE COOKING

Use cooking methods that lock in the vitamins and minerals needed for healthy bones to make sure your meals are nutrient-dense. Steaming is one of the best ways to do this, especially with veggies, as it uses less water and short cooking times to lock in the vitamins that are soluble in water, like B vitamins and vitamin C. It's also important to avoid overcooking and to cover the food to keep the steam and heat contained.

While boiling can lose nutrients in the water, roasting vegetables or proteins like chicken and fish can enhance flavors without losing nutrients. To avoid nutrient loss from direct exposure to high heat, use parchment paper or a baking dish with a lid. Baking or roasting is another efficient method that uses dry heat to cook food evenly and retain most of its nutrients.

When done correctly, microwave cooking can also be a nutrient-preserving technique. By cooking proteins and vegetables quickly and using little water, you can shorten the cooking time and preserve more vitamins and minerals. When microwaving, make sure to cut the food into uniform pieces to ensure even cooking and preservation of nutrients.

COOKING WITH VERY LITTLE SALT ADDED

Cutting back on salt can help maintain bone health because too much sodium can cause calcium loss. To cook with less salt, begin with whole, fresh ingredients, which are naturally lower in sodium than processed foods. Instead of using a salt shaker, add flavor to your food with herbs, spices, and citrus juices.

Cooking methods that bring out the rich, natural tastes of meats and vegetables and enhance their flavor without adding extra salt include roasting, grilling, and slow cooking. Roasting vegetables with a drizzle of olive oil and a sprinkle of herbs like rosemary or thyme, for example, can produce a tasty, savory dish without adding extra sodium.

Use sea salt or kosher salt, which has larger crystals and can provide more flavor with less quantity; taste your food before adding more salt to prevent over-seasoning; and use salt sparingly and strategically, adding a small amount at the end of cooking to maximize the flavor impact with less sodium.

INCLUDING SPICES AND BONE-FRIENDLY HERBS

Incorporating bone-friendly herbs like parsley, sage, and dill can provide essential nutrients like vitamin K, which is crucial for bone health. Fresh herbs can be sprinkled over dishes right before serving to preserve their vitamins and add a burst of fresh flavor. Herbs and spices are a great way to enhance the flavor and nutritional profile of your meals.

Ginger and turmeric are two examples of spices with anti-inflammatory qualities that can support bone health.

Turmeric, in particular, contains curcumin, which has been demonstrated to help reduce bone loss. You can use ginger fresh or as a powder in marinades, stir-fries, and baked goods. Add turmeric to soups, stews, and curries, or blend it into smoothies for a nutritious boost.

Try blending herbs and spices to create flavor combinations that you like. For example, combine thyme and rosemary to roast chicken or cilantro and lime to make a zesty marinade for fish.

These combinations not only improve flavor but also add extra nutrients that support bone health overall.

HEALTHY ALTERNATIVES TO CUSTOMARY RECIPES

Replace refined grains with whole grains, such as quinoa, brown rice, or whole wheat pasta, which offer more fiber, vitamins, and minerals; for example, replace white rice in a stir-fry with quinoa, or use whole grain pasta in your favorite pasta dishes, to create bone-friendly meals without sacrificing flavor.

For those who are lactose intolerant or prefer plant-based options, dairy substitutes can also be helpful. Almond milk, fortified with calcium and vitamin D, can be substituted for cow's milk in smoothies, soups, and baked goods. Nutritional yeast can be used as a good source of B vitamins and as a cheesy substitute in sauces and casseroles.

To improve the nutritional value of your meals and support bone health, replace unhealthy fats with healthier options like olive oil, avocado, or nut butter. You can also use mashed avocado instead of butter on toast or as a spread in sandwiches. Greek yogurt can be used in place of mayonnaise in dressings and dips to increase protein and decrease unhealthy fats.

ADVICE FOR PLANNING AND PREPARING MEALS

Easier maintenance of a bone-healthy diet can be achieved through efficient meal preparation and planning. Begin by organizing your meals into a weekly schedule that incorporates a range of foods that are good for your bones, such as leafy greens, nuts, seeds, and lean proteins. Making your meals ahead of time guarantees that you have everything you need and helps you avoid making unhealthy decisions at the last minute.

Make large batches of soups, stews, and casseroles that can be portioned out and frozen for later use. This method not only simplifies your weeknight dinners but also helps you control portion sizes and reduce food waste. Batch cooking can save time and guarantee you always have wholesome meals on hand.

Frozen veggies can be just as nutritious as fresh ones and are convenient for quick meals. Keep your pantry stocked with essentials like whole grains, legumes, and healthy oils, so you're always ready to cook up a bone-healthy meal. Include a combination of fresh and frozen produce in your meal plan to ensure you have a constant supply of nutrient-dense ingredients.

CHAPTER SIX

MEAL PLANNING: BREAKFAST RECIPES

BREAKFAST IDEAS HIGH IN CALCIUM

A bowl of yogurt topped with fresh fruit, such as berries, and a sprinkle of almonds can help support strong bones and lower the risk of osteoporosis. Yogurt is a great source of calcium, and adding fruits and nuts to it provides vitamins and antioxidants, while almonds add an extra boost of calcium and healthy fats. Another option is to make a smoothie with calcium-fortified orange juice, spinach, and a banana for sweetness. This smoothie is creamy, nutrient-dense, easy to make, and full of bone-strengthening properties.

A delicious and satisfying breakfast option that is high in calcium is a tofu scramble, which is made with tofu, garlic, turmeric, and your favorite vegetables like bell peppers, spinach, and tomatoes. Once the tofu and veggies are tender and flavorful, they can be cooked in a skillet with a side order of whole-grain toast, which often contains added calcium. For a sweet option, try overnight oats made with calcium-fortified milk or plant-based milk. Combine rolled oats, chia seeds, a splash of vanilla, and your choice of milk; let it sit overnight. In the morning, top with sliced fruits and a drizzle of honey for a delicious and nutritious breakfast.

RECIPES ENHANCED WITH VITAMIN D

A good way to make sure you get enough vitamin D for breakfast is to have fortified cereal with milk. A lot of breakfast cereals come fortified with vitamin D, and when you pair them with milk (which is also fortified), you get a double dose of this essential nutrient. You can also top your cereal with some sliced bananas or berries for extra flavor and nutrition. Lastly, you can make scrambled eggs with fortified mushrooms. You can sauté mushrooms in buttermilk to boost their vitamin D content, and when combined with eggs, they make a delicious and nourishing breakfast dish.

If you'd rather have something savory, consider preparing a breakfast burrito with fortified ingredients.

Toast whole-grain tortillas, and top with scrambled eggs, black beans, avocado, and a sprinkle of cheese (black beans are high in protein and fiber, and cheese when fortified, adds extra vitamin D). Serve with salsa for a tasty and vitamin D-rich breakfast.

If you'd rather have a smoothie, blend fortified orange juice with frozen mango, a handful of spinach, and a scoop of yogurt. This vitamin-rich beverage is perfect for a quick and nourishing morning meal.

IDEAS FOR HIGH-PROTEIN BREAKFASTS

A classic breakfast of eggs and avocado gets you started each day. Eggs are a fantastic source of high-quality protein and can be prepared in a variety of ways, such as scrambled, boiled, or poached. Pair them with half an avocado for healthy fats and a satisfying, protein-rich meal. You can also add a slice of whole-grain toast for extra fiber and nutrients. Greek yogurt parfaits are another high-protein breakfast option. Greek yogurt is higher in protein than regular yogurt and when layered with granola and fresh fruits, they make a tasty and nutritious meal that's simple to prepare and enjoy.

Quinoa is a complete protein, which means it contains all nine essential amino acids, making it a great option for a high-protein meal. Cook the quinoa according to the package instructions and combine it with sautéed vegetables like spinach, bell peppers, and tomatoes. Top with a poached egg for a creamy texture and an extra protein boost. If you're on the go, protein smoothies are a great option. Blend protein powder, almond milk, frozen berries, and a handful of spinach to create a high-protein, high-nutrient smoothie that will keep you full and energized throughout the morning.

FIBER-PRICH BREAKFAST OPTIONS

A smoothie bowl made with blended fruits and vegetables is another healthy option that is high in fiber. Use a base of spinach or kale, add a banana for sweetness, blend with almond milk, and top with chia seeds, flaxseeds, and granola for a crunchy, high-fiber breakfast.

Oats are a great source of soluble fiber, which can help lower cholesterol levels and improve heart health. Cook the oats with milk or water and add toppings like sliced bananas, berries, and a handful of walnuts or almonds for extra fiber and nutrients. Another fiber-rich option is a smoothie bowl made with blended fruits and vegetables.

Another option is to have whole-grain toast with avocado and tomato. The high fiber content of whole-grain bread pairs well with mashed avocado and sliced tomatoes to create a tasty and nutritious meal. A little salt and pepper can enhance the flavor. For a more involved breakfast, try a vegetable frittata. Simply whisk together eggs, and chopped veggies (such as broccoli, bell peppers, and onions), and bake in the oven until cooked. The combination of veggies and eggs creates a well-balanced and satisfying meal that tastes great.

SIMPLE AND FAST BREAKFAST RECIPES

Having quick and easy breakfast options is important because mornings can be hectic. A simple yet nutritious breakfast option is smoothies, which you can make by blending your favorite fruits, spinach, protein powder, and almond milk. Smoothies are easy to make and convenient to carry on the go. Another quick breakfast option is overnight oats, which you can make by combining rolled oats, chia seeds, milk or yogurt, and a little honey in a jar. The next morning, you can serve this ready-to-eat meal with fresh fruits and nuts on top.

Consider a breakfast wrap. Use a whole-grain tortilla and fill it with scrambled eggs, black beans, spinach, and avocado. Wrap it up and enjoy a nutritious and easy breakfast that's packed with protein, fiber, and healthy fats. These quick and easy recipes ensure you start your day with a balanced meal, even on the busiest mornings. Beat eggs, a splash of milk, and your choice of chopped vegetables and cheese. Pour the mixture into a muffin tin and bake until the eggs are set. You can make these egg muffins ahead of time and store them in the refrigerator for an easy grab-and-go breakfast.

HEALTHY SALADS AND THEIR INGREDIENTS

Healthy salads are a vital component of an osteoporosis diet because they provide a range of vitamins and minerals that are important for strong bones. Start with a base of calcium- and vitamin K-rich leafy greens, such as spinach, kale, or arugula.

Then, add vibrant vegetables, like bell peppers, carrots, and tomatoes, to supply a variety of antioxidants and phytonutrients. Finally, add fruits, like berries, oranges, or apples, for a little sweetness and an additional vitamin boost.

Lean protein options, like grilled chicken, turkey, or tofu, help maintain muscle mass and promote overall health. Beans and legumes, like lentils or chickpeas, are great plant-based sources of protein and give your salad a satisfying texture. Nuts and seeds, like sunflower, chia, or almond, add crunch and healthy fats and protein to your salad.

For added taste and nutrition, try dressings made with healthy oils like avocado or olive oil mixed with vinegar or lemon juice; fresh herbs like basil, cilantro, or parsley can add flavor and nutrients; with these ingredients, making a balanced, bone-friendly salad is fun and easy to put together and guarantees a nutrient-dense meal that promotes bone health.

STEWS & SOUPS TO BUILD BONES

A satisfying and nutrient-dense lunch option, bone-building soups and stews are particularly helpful for people with osteoporosis. Begin with a base of bone broth, which is high in collagen and minerals that promote bone health.

Add a variety of vegetables, like carrots, celery, onions, and garlic, which supply important vitamins and minerals. You can add leafy greens, like spinach or kale, toward the end of cooking to preserve the nutrients.

Lean meats—such as chicken, turkey, or fish—are essential for maintaining bone health and muscle mass.

If you'd rather go plant-based, consider beans, lentils, or tofu—all of which are high in fiber and protein. Whole grains—like barley, quinoa, or brown rice—can be added to the stew to increase its nutritional value and fillingness while also adding extra minerals like phosphorus and magnesium.

Spices and herbs such as turmeric, ginger, rosemary, or thyme can be used to season soups and stews; these additions not only improve flavor but also have anti-inflammatory properties. Slow cooking releases the nutrients and creates a flavorful, filling meal that is good for bone density and general health.

IDEAS FOR WHOLE GRAIN LUNCHES

While quinoa is a complete protein and offers a good balance of amino acids necessary for bone repair, it also makes a light yet satisfying lunch option. Whole grains are a great addition to a lunch menu aimed at supporting bone health. They are rich in essential nutrients like magnesium, phosphorus, and fiber, which contribute to overall wellness and bone strength.

Another flexible option is to make brown rice bowls, which you can top with steamed or sautéed vegetables, lean proteins like grilled chicken or tofu, and a little low-sodium soy sauce or teriyaki for a filling and healthy meal. Brown rice is high in fiber and complex carbohydrates, which help release energy slowly.

If you're feeling daring, consider making a stir-fry of barley and colorful veggies like bell peppers, broccoli, and snap peas.

To bring out the flavor of the barley, add some garlic, ginger, and a sprinkling of sesame oil. This dish is a good source of vitamins, minerals, and antioxidants that help support bone health.

LUNCHTIME SOURCES OF LEAN PROTEIN

For lunch, you should include a lean protein source that will help you maintain muscle mass and support bone health. One popular and adaptable option is grilled chicken breast, which can be sliced and added to salads, mixed with whole grains like quinoa or brown rice, or used in wraps with lots of fresh vegetables. Chicken is high in protein and provides essential amino acids that are necessary for bone maintenance and repair.

Another great source of lean protein is fish. Fish that has been baked or grilled goes well with steamed vegetables and whole grains like brown rice or quinoa. Choices like salmon, tuna, or cod are not only high in protein but also contain omega-3 fatty acids, which have anti-inflammatory qualities and support bone health.

If you'd rather eat plant-based foods, tofu and tempeh are excellent options. Both are high in calcium and can be easily added to a variety of dishes.

For example, tofu can be stir-fried with vegetables and whole grains, while tempeh can be marinated and grilled to make a substantial salad or sandwich topping. Either way, these soy-based proteins guarantee a high-protein meal that promotes bone and muscle health.

For both overall health and bone health, lunch meals should be well-balanced. To begin, make sure each meal has a range of nutrients from various food groups. Pair lean proteins, like turkey, grilled chicken, or tofu, with a generous amount of vegetables, like broccoli, bell peppers, and leafy greens. These vegetables offer important vitamins and minerals, like calcium and vitamin K, which are vital for bone health.

A well-rounded and nutrient-dense meal can be achieved by including whole grains such as quinoa, brown rice, or whole wheat pasta, which are rich in fiber and complex carbohydrates. Whole grains are also a good source of important nutrients, such as phosphorus and magnesium, which support bone density.

Don't forget about healthy fats, which you can get from foods like avocado, nuts, and seeds.

DINNER OPTIONS HIGH IN CALCIUM

Developing dinner options that are high in calcium can be tasty and helpful for people who are trying to build stronger bones. To begin, make a hearty stir-fry of spinach and tofu, as spinach is high in calcium and tofu adds even more calcium to the dish. Sauté fresh spinach in olive oil, then add cubed tofu and a little soy sauce. Cook until the tofu is lightly browned and the spinach is wilted. Serve this over quinoa or brown rice to finish the meal with a high-fiber, nutrient-dense foundation.

Another delicious and calcium-rich dinner option is baked salmon served with steamed broccoli. Salmon is high in calcium and also contains vitamin D, which is essential for calcium absorption. Before baking the salmon, season it with herbs, garlic, and lemon. To season the broccoli, simply steam it until it is tender and add a small amount of sea salt and olive oil. Either way, you can be sure you're eating a well-balanced, flavorful meal that promotes bone health.

In a big pot, sauté onions and garlic in olive oil, then add chopped kale and canned white beans. Pour in vegetable broth and simmer until the kale is tender. Finish with a splash of almond milk to give the soup a creamy texture without adding dairy, making it perfect for those who are lactose intolerant. Kale is a powerhouse of calcium, and white beans add protein and additional calcium.

ONE-POT DINNERS FOR EASE

A classic option for busy weeknights is a one-pot meal: brown chicken pieces in a large pot, then add chopped carrots, celery, potatoes, and onions. Pour in chicken broth and season with bay leaves and thyme. Simmer until the chicken is cooked through and the vegetables are tender. This filling stew not only saves time but also provides a powerful nutritional boost with a variety of vitamins and minerals.

Quinoa and vegetable paella is a Mediterranean-style one-pot dish. Start by sautéing the garlic, onions, and bell peppers in olive oil.

Then, add the quinoa, diced tomatoes, and vegetable broth. For added flavor, add a pinch of saffron and smoked paprika. Towards the end of cooking, stir in the peas and artichoke hearts. This dish is colorful and flavorful, and it's also high in plant-based protein and fiber, making it a healthy dinner option.

Try a lentil and sweet potato curry for a filling but healthful option. First, sauté onions, garlic, and ginger in a large pot. Next, add cubed sweet potatoes and lentils. Finally, pour in coconut milk and vegetable broth, along with curry powder and turmeric. Simmer until the curry is thick and fragrant and the lentils and sweet potatoes are tender. Serve the curry over brown rice or with naan bread for a complete, nutritious meal that's quick to make.

IDEAS FOR VEGETARIAN AND VEGAN DINNERS

Dinners made without meat can be filling and nutritious. One such dish is stuffed bell peppers, which are filled with quinoa, black beans, corn, and diced tomatoes and seasoned with cumin and chili powder.

The filled peppers are baked until they are soft and the filling is heated through. This dish is visually appealing and full of protein and fiber, making it a hearty alternative to meat.

A curry made with chickpeas and fresh spinach is another fantastic idea. In a large pot, sauté the onions, garlic, and ginger. Add the chickpeas and fresh spinach. Pour in the coconut milk and season with the curry powder, cumin, and coriander. Simmer until the spinach wilts and the flavors combine. Serve the curry over brown rice or with flatbread on the side for a plant-based protein and iron-rich meal that's perfect for a vegetarian or vegan diet.

A creamy avocado pasta can make a delicious dinner for a pasta lover. Cook your preferred pasta according to the directions on the package. In the meantime, pure ripe avocados with garlic, fresh basil, lemon juice, and a small amount of olive oil until smooth. Toss the cooked pasta with the avocado sauce, then top with baby spinach and cherry tomatoes for flavor and nutrients.

This dish is high in nutrients and low in fat, making it a great option for a vegan dinner.

RECIPES FOR SEAFOOD HIGH IN OMEGA-3S

Omega-3-rich seafood can help maintain bone health and general well-being. Here's a simple but delicious recipe for grilled salmon with a lemon-dill sauce: season salmon fillets with salt, pepper, and olive oil; grill until cooked through; for the sauce, combine Greek yogurt, lemon juice, fresh dill, and a dash of garlic powder. This dish pairs well with steamed asparagus or a mixed green salad.

A quick and healthy omega-3-rich dinner option is to stir-fry shrimp and vegetables in a large skillet with olive oil until the shrimp are pink and cooked through, then set aside. In the same skillet, add a mixture of your favorite vegetables, like bell peppers, carrots, and snap peas, and stir-fry until the vegetables are tender-crisp. Finally, return the shrimp to the skillet and season with a little soy sauce and sesame seeds. Serve the shrimp and vegetable stir-fry over brown rice or noodles.

A seafood chowder is a filling and hearty dish that can be made by sautéing onions, celery, and garlic in butter in a large pot. Then, add diced potatoes, fish stock, and a combination of your favorite seafood, like clams, cod, and shrimp. Simmer until the potatoes are soft and the seafood is cooked through. Finally, stir in some cream for richness and season with bay leaves and thyme. This chowder is a great way to spend a chilly evening and is a good source of protein and omega-3 fatty acids.

DINNER RECIPES THAT STRENGTHEN BONES

Beef is a great source of protein and minerals like zinc and iron, which are essential for bone health. Brown beef chunks in a pot, then add chopped carrots, potatoes, and celery. Pour in beef broth and season with rosemary and thyme. Simmer until the beef is tender and the vegetables are cooked through. This filling stew is packed with nutrients that support strong bones. It's a great way to start a dinner that promotes bone strength.

This dish, which combines lean protein from the chicken with calcium from the cheese and broccoli, is delicious for bone health. To make it, layer cooked chicken breasts and steamed broccoli in a baking dish. Top with a mixture of shredded cheese and whole-grain breadcrumbs. Bake in the oven until the cheese is melted and bubbly.

An excellent plant-based option would be a tofu and kale stir-fry. Tofu is a great source of calcium, and kale is high in vitamin K, which is important for healthy bones. Heat tofu cubes until golden brown in a large skillet, then add chopped kale and garlic; stir-fry until the kale is tender and wilted. Season with a little soy sauce and sesame seeds. Serve over brown rice or quinoa for a hearty and nutritious meal that will strengthen bones.

IDEAS FOR NUTRIENT-DENSE SNACKS

Finding nutrient-dense snack options is essential for preserving bone health. Choosing vitamin and mineral-rich snacks supports bone density and overall strength. Snacking on Greek yogurt with mixed berries and almonds is a great option because it offers a powerful combination of calcium, vitamin D, and protein that is necessary for bone health. Hummus with carrot and cucumber sticks is another excellent option because it provides a combination of calcium, magnesium, and vitamin K that supports bone mineralization and maintenance. Finally, a handful of nuts and seeds, like almonds, chia seeds, and pumpkin seeds, is a great way to satisfy cravings while also supporting bone health and lowering the risk of osteoporosis.

SNACKS HIGH IN CALCIUM

Including calcium-rich snacks in your diet is vital for strong bones. Choose from snacks like cheese and whole-grain crackers, which offer a significant amount of calcium required for bone mineralization and strength. You can also enjoy sardines with bones, which are a great source of calcium, vitamin D, and omega-3 fatty acids, all of which are important for bone health. Another excellent option is to combine a calcium-fortified granola bar with fortified soy or almond milk, which provides a dual dose of calcium and vitamin D for maximum bone support. By incorporating these calcium-rich snacks into your daily routine, you can be sure to meet your dietary calcium requirements, supporting bone density and lowering the risk of fractures linked to osteoporosis. Regularly enjoying these snacks not only helps.

BONE-FRIENDLY DESSERT DISHES THAT ARE HEALTHY

Making bone-friendly desserts lets you enjoy while maintaining the health of your bones. For example, a yogurt parfait with fresh fruit and granola combines calcium-rich yogurt with antioxidant-rich fruits and whole grains that support bone strength.

Baked apples with walnuts and cinnamon are a delicious option that provides a combination of calcium, potassium, and vitamin C that helps with bone mineralization and maintenance. Chia seed pudding, made with fortified almond milk and topped with berries, is a rich treat that contains the essential nutrients for bone health—ozone-3 fatty acids, calcium, and vitamin D. These desserts not only satiate your sweet tooth but also add to your daily intake of nutrients, supporting strong and healthy bones when consumed.

SMOOTHIES AND THEIR ADVANTAGES FOR BONE HEALTH

Smoothies that contain ingredients like spinach, kale, and yogurt, which are high in calcium, vitamin K, and magnesium, which are essential for maintaining bone density and strength, can be blended with fruits like bananas and oranges to provide vitamin C, which promotes collagen formation, which is crucial for bone structure.

Almond butter or chia seeds, which are high in omega-3 fatty acids, can also be added to smoothies to support overall bone health and reduce inflammation.

These nutrient-dense smoothies are not only a refreshing way to consume nutrients that are good for your bones, but they also contribute to overall well-being when consumed regularly.

SNACKS AND DESSERTS CREATED AT HOME TO STRENGTHEN BONES

The secret to maintaining optimal bone health is to make homemade snacks and desserts that support bone strength. For example, you can make kale chips seasoned with calcium-rich nutritional yeast, which is a savory treat packed with vitamin K and magnesium essential for bone mineralization.

Another delicious option is to make your trail mix with dried fruits and nuts, which provides a mix of calcium, potassium, and vitamin D that supports bone density.

For dessert, you can bake oatmeal cookies with dried figs and flaxseeds, which offer a healthy dose of fiber, calcium, and omega-3 fatty acids that are beneficial for bone health. By making these homemade treats, you can ensure that you get the essential nutrients you need to maintain strong and healthy bones.

CHAPTER SEVEN

PARTICULAR THOUGHTS AND ADJUSTMENTS

DIETARY MODIFICATIONS FOR VARIOUS AGE GROUPS

To effectively manage osteoporosis through diet, it is important to customize nutritional strategies for each age group. For example, younger adults should prioritize building peak bone mass by emphasizing foods high in calcium, such as dairy products, fortified cereals, and leafy greens.

They should also ensure that they get enough vitamin D to facilitate calcium absorption, which can be achieved through exposure to sunlight, fortified foods, or supplements. Middle-aged adults should balance their calcium intake with sufficient protein and micronutrients from a variety of sources, such as lean meats, nuts, and whole grains. Finally, weight-bearing exercises should be incorporated to complement dietary efforts and promote bone density and strength.

Seniors need to make dietary adjustments to prevent bone loss. Eating more calcium-rich foods is still important, but if dietary intake is low, there should be an increased focus on supplements. Vitamin D is even more important because skin synthesis and absorption efficiency are decreased, so regular supplementation and dietary inclusion are required. Protein consumption should be maintained to support bone and muscle health, along with ongoing weight-bearing exercises and activities that improve balance and coordination. By customizing dietary strategies to different age groups, people can effectively manage osteoporosis risk and maintain bone health throughout their lives.

HANDLING OTHER MEDICAL CONDITIONS IN ADDITION TO OSTEOPOROSIS

Handling osteoporosis in conjunction with other medical conditions necessitates carefully thought-out dietary approaches that promote general health while catering to individual requirements. For diabetics, stable blood sugar levels must be maintained, which can be accomplished with a balanced diet full of whole grains, lean meats, and non-starchy vegetables. Calcium consumption must be watched, with low-fat dairy products or fortified substitutes to support bone health without interfering with diabetes management. Adequate hydration is also critical, supporting kidney function and bone mineralization while reducing the risk of dehydration, which can aggravate both conditions.

Vitamin D supplementation may be necessary due to potential malabsorption issues, ensuring optimal bone health support. Managing medications that affect bone metabolism, such as corticosteroids, with calcium and vitamin D supplementation becomes crucial, requiring close monitoring and adjustment by healthcare providers to effectively mitigate osteoporosis risk. For individuals with gastrointestinal conditions like Crohn's disease or celiac disease, nutrient absorption may be compromised, necessitating adjustments to the osteoporosis diet.

Managing eating out while following an osteoporosis diet requires making thoughtful decisions to preserve bone health without compromising social dining experiences. Selecting eateries that serve nutrient-dense dishes like grilled fish, leafy greens, and calcium-fortified options helps satisfy dietary requirements when having meals away from home. Asking for adjustments or substitutions, like steamed vegetables instead of fried ones, lowers excess sodium and preserves nutrient density. Selecting nutrient-dense appetizers like yogurt-based dips or cheese salads offers a healthy beginning to the meal, supporting bone health through a diverse range of dietary choices.

Portion control and choosing lean protein sources such as chicken or beans, along with whole grains or quinoa as side dishes, increase meal satisfaction and nutritional value when eating out. Reducing alcohol and choosing water or calcium-fortified beverages when dining out further supports bone health goals.

People can enjoy eating out while making dietary choices that support bone density and overall well-being by making advance plans and looking over menus for osteoporosis-friendly options.

MODIFYING RECIPES TO MEET DIETARY REQUIREMENTS

Recipes can be modified to meet dietary needs while adhering to osteoporosis-friendly principles by using inventive substitutions and thoughtful ingredient selection. For those who are lactose intolerant, selecting lactose-free dairy products or fortified non-dairy alternatives guarantees enough calcium intake without causing discomfort in the digestive tract. Adding calcium-rich vegetables, such as broccoli or kale, to recipes promotes bone health objectives and adds nutritional value. Using herbs and spices to add flavor reduces the need for excessive salt, which is good for heart health and bone density maintenance.

Those who follow a gluten-free diet because they have celiac disease or are sensitive to gluten should use gluten-free grains like quinoa or brown rice as the basis for recipes. This will support nutrient diversity and digestive health. Adding sources of vitamin D, like fortified cereals or mushrooms, guarantees comprehensive bone health support without compromising dietary restrictions. Changing recipes to include lean proteins, like tofu or legumes, and adding omega-3-rich foods, like flaxseeds or walnuts, will further improve nutritional balance and bone density maintenance. People can enjoy tasty and varied meals while adhering to their osteoporosis diet goals by modifying recipes and choosing ingredients carefully.

FAQS AND COMMON QUESTIONS REGARDING SPECIAL DIETARY NEEDS

Answering frequently asked questions and addressing common concerns about special dietary needs related to osteoporosis enables people to make educated decisions that effectively support bone health. A lot of people question whether supplements, such as calcium and vitamin D, are really necessary. It's important to stress that although dietary sources are ideal, supplements guarantee consistent intake, particularly in cases of dietary limitations or inadequate absorption. Dairy intake is a common concern, especially when it comes to lactose intolerance or vegan preferences. Emphasizing alternative calcium sources like fortified non-dairy milk, leafy greens, and canned fish with bones reassures people about the variety of dietary options that support bone health.

Controlling sodium consumption is another common concern because too much salt can lead to bone loss. Promoting the use of herbs, spices, and citrus flavors in cooking improves flavor without compromising bone health, supporting heart health at the same time. Recognizing the importance of protein in bone maintenance is critical because lean meats, legumes, and nuts provide essential nutrients for bone density and muscle support. Dispelling myths about dietary fats and stressing the importance of healthy fats from sources like avocados or olive oil promotes overall well-being while supporting bone health objectives.

CHAPTER EIGHT

SUSTAINING BONE HEALTH OVER TIME

REGULAR PHYSICAL ACTIVITY IS ESSENTIAL

Frequent exercise is essential for maintaining and improving bone health, and it is especially important for those who are managing osteoporosis. Weight-bearing exercises, such as walking, jogging, dancing, or strength training, stimulate bone formation and lower the risk of fractures. These exercises put stress on bones, which causes them to become stronger and denser over time. Diverse exercises that target different muscle groups and bones are necessary to ensure comprehensive benefits for bone health. Beginners should begin with low-impact exercises and work their way up to more intense ones as their fitness increases.

Setting realistic goals and creating a routine are essential for incorporating physical activity into daily life. Maintaining consistency is also essential for long-term benefits, like better posture, balance, and general well-being. Speaking with a healthcare provider or fitness expert can help customize an exercise plan that meets specific needs and ensures safe progression. Tracking progress and making necessary adjustments to routines ensures continued motivation and optimal bone health outcomes.

KEEPING AN EYE ON BONE HEALTH AND DENSITY

Bone density tests, such as dual-energy X-ray absorptiometry (DEXA) scans, assess bone strength and density levels; they provide valuable information on bone mineral content and help healthcare providers evaluate fracture risk. Regular screenings are recommended, especially for postmenopausal women and older adults, to detect changes in bone density early and intervene promptly. Monitoring bone density and health is fundamental for individuals with osteoporosis to track progress and make informed decisions about treatment and lifestyle adjustments.

Apart from bone density tests, other health indicators like calcium and vitamin D levels and other bone health markers should also be monitored. Knowing the outcomes of these tests enables people to work with healthcare professionals to create customized plans to maintain bone density and lower the risk of fracture. Lifestyle changes, such as dietary changes and physical activity schedules, can be adjusted based on continuous monitoring, guaranteeing proactive management of osteoporosis.

LIFESTYLE SUGGESTIONS FOR STRONG BONES

The best way to manage osteoporosis is to adopt lifestyle practices that support bone strength. Avoiding smoking and excessive alcohol consumption is also important because these habits weaken bones and increase the risk of fracture. Making sure you get enough calcium and vitamin D from your diet and supplements supports bone mineralization and density. Foods high in calcium include dairy products, leafy greens, and fortified foods.

A healthy body weight is maintained by eating a balanced diet and exercising regularly.

This helps to maintain bone mass and minimizes stress on joints. Weight-bearing exercises and resistance training strengthen bones and improve muscle strength and flexibility, both of which are important for maintaining overall bone health. Balance and posture exercises also help to improve stability and lower the risk of falls, which can result in fractures, especially in those who have osteoporosis.

INCLUDING THE OSTEOPOROSIS DIET IN EVERYDAY ACTIVITIES

A registered dietitian can help customize meal plans and ensure nutritional adequacy. Including sources of vitamin D, such as fatty fish, egg yolks, and fortified cereals, improves calcium absorption and contributes to bone strength. Following an osteoporosis diet entails making strategic dietary choices that support bone health and overall well-being. Stressing calcium-rich foods, such as dairy products, leafy greens, and fortified foods, ensures adequate calcium intake necessary for bone mineralization.

A balanced diet that includes whole grains, fruits, vegetables, lean proteins, and low amounts of sodium and caffeine can help maintain calcium levels in the body and lower the risk of bone loss. Hydration is also essential for maintaining optimal bone health because it supports waste removal and nutrient transport, which in turn helps maintain overall bone density. These nutrients, in addition to calcium and vitamin D, are critical for bone health and overall vitality.

SOURCES OF CONTINUED ASSISTANCE AND KNOWLEDGE

Individuals with osteoporosis are better equipped to make decisions about their health and well-being when they have access to trustworthy resources for ongoing support and information. Healthcare professionals, such as primary care physicians, orthopedists, and endocrinologists who specialize in bone health, can provide expert guidance on treatment options, lifestyle changes, and preventive measures. Patient advocacy organizations and support groups can also be valuable sources of peer support, educational materials, and opportunities for community engagement for those managing osteoporosis.

Online resources and credible bone health websites provide extensive information on managing osteoporosis, dietary advice, exercise protocols, and the most recent research findings. Educational materials, webinars, and virtual seminars can be accessed to increase awareness of bone health and encourage proactive health management. Speaking with medical professionals and taking part in educational events guarantee continuous learning and enable people to effectively advocate for their needs related to bone health.

www.ingramcontent.com/pod-product-compliance
Lightning Source LLC
Chambersburg PA
CBHW061300250726
48653CB00002B/707